OVERTIRED?
OVERWEIGHT?

OVERTIRED?
OVERWEIGHT?
THE SOLUTION

PETER TAYLOR

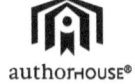

authorHOUSE®

AuthorHouse™
1663 Liberty Drive
Bloomington, IN 47403
www.authorhouse.com
Phone: 1-800-839-8640

Published by AuthorHouse   02/21/2013

ISBN: 978-1-4817-8214-2 (sc)
ISBN: 978-1-4817-8213-5 (e)

Contents

Foreword

This booklet is the culmination of years of practising as a therapist and experiencing the heartache of so many clients who have found their lives blighted by fatigue. It seems to be such an enormous problem worldwide but is seen as normal and therefore not as a disorder. Why governments and health services do not invest more money in combating this problem is a mystery, so I decided to add a little information that I hope will help those who read this.

However, this information is science based and is therefore technical which means it requires a little patience to read.

Your body is unbelievably remarkable. An absolute miracle. By reading this booklet you will give it a fighting chance to give back to you the energy you have lost and for you to find the weight you wish for.

Introduction

Peter Taylor came from a background of management, commerce and marketing.

Whilst developing a health-spa in Devon, UK, he became an alternative therapist and learned the importance of looking at life in many ways. His experience has enabled him to combine all the various therapies he has learnt along the way into a package that really can have a positive effect upon people with health problems.

He sees a lot of tired and sometimes obese people and is able to help because of his knowledge of nutrition, of what it is that we eat, and what it is that makes us so tired.

This booklet is all that is required to gain energy and maybe lose weight. There is no magic wand. There are no short cuts. There is no easy way. Only hard work and determination coupled with the knowledge that this booklet provides.

Chapter One

Background

This booklet is totally uncompromising. It is based upon fact. It tells you what you need to know and what you ought to know but not necessarily what you want to know, so be prepared for some home truths.

There are many diets, and I expect you have been on one or more of them. If you thought they worked you would not be reading this. You may already have spent shedloads of money only to find out that they do not.

There are no short cuts to finding extra energy and losing weight. In a world where we are always seeking easier ways of doing things, this is really hard to take. But believe me, there really are no short cuts.

Only you can rediscover your energy. Remember the days when you were a child? All that energy? No one else can do this for you, but if you follow my suggestions it will not take long before you feel the benefits.

So where do we start?

A little background reading is helpful

There are only two types of people wishing to rediscover their lost energy and lose weight.

    A) Those who do not know the difference between a calorie-rich and a calorie-poor diet and the difference between slow-release and rapid-release carbohydrates.

    B) Those who do know the difference but cannot bring themselves to make the sacrifice.

These people are not in control of their own eating. They do not need technical advice but need help and encouragement to carry out plans that they are able to cope with.

This booklet will help people from both categories.

This technical information regarding energy loss is relatively simple, so read on. The daily consumption of calories minus the daily burning of calories equals the amount of calories remaining in the body. Calories equal energy, but if not used, excess calories will convert to excess weight and create weight gain. This energy comes in two packets: slow-release energy and rapid-release energy.

Rapid-release energy comes from processed carbohydrates, such as processed sugar, white rice and wheat or white flour and is found in bread, rolls, pizzas, quiches, pasta, muffins, biscuits, cakes, couscous, sweets, milk and so on.

The glucose from the gluten in the processed wheat is rapidly absorbed into the cells for storage and unless burned off quite quickly will become extra fat.

Slow-release energy comes from unprocessed wheat or brown rice, millet, rye, barley, root vegetables and other carbohydrates and takes much longer to become easily-absorbed glucose. This is because it contains the germ, which itself contains nutrients, such as vitamins and minerals and also the fibre, which is the outside covering or husk. These two components of a grain take much more time to digest, thereby releasing glucose from the gluten more slowly. As we burn calories all the time, even when not exercising, the smaller amount of glucose from slow-release carbohydrates is burned almost as soon as it is absorbed, so much less gets stored in fat cells.

The problem lies in rapid-release carbohydrates. Because much of the germ and fibre are removed in the processing of the grain, all the glucose contained in the gluten is released at once from the digestive system much more rapidly into the blood stream and cells.

Whilst this enables us to feel energised rapidly, it is dangerous to have too much glucose in the blood at any one time. Insulin is pumped into the blood stream so that the glucose can be absorbed into the cells, either for instant use or for storage in a fat cell.

The problem is increased because with so much insulin available the glucose is absorbed rapidly, leaving the blood deficient of glucose, which means you feel tired. When you feel tired, you seek more glucose, repeating the cycle and so you go through the day in peaks and troughs of energy and fatigue.

Everyone has different rates of burning calories and everyone has different rates of absorbing calories. Some people just have to work harder at staying slim because of the way their mother and father designed them. Excess calories will lead to excess fat. Rapid-release carbohydrates lead to peaks and troughs of energy. When you feel tired, you tend to eat to replenish lost energy. Unless what you eat satisfies your hunger, you will continue to eat, which just adds calories. It becomes a downward spiral into becoming tired and overweight.

One of the most difficult things to contend with is metabolism. Metabolism is the rate at which your cells function. All cells need oxygen as a fuel, so cells with a high metabolic rate will burn more calories. The problem with excess fat cells is that their metabolism is slow, so much more activity is required to burn off their calories.

Add to this rather depressing news the fact that we are all born with billions of fat cells which simply store fat. These cells are able to stretch so that they can contain lots of fat. But when they are full, the body makes more cells to store fat. You can have a body with billions more fat cells than when you first started your life.

The problem with this increase in fat cells is that when you start to lose weight, the number of fat cells will always remain the same. All that happens is that the amount of fat in each cell is reduced. It is much easier for a slim person to lose weight because they have fewer fat cells. It's easier to lose fat from one billion cells than two billion cells. Losing weight is harder the the more fat cells you have.

Chapter Two

It's easy to get fatigued

If domestic animals are fed highly attractive food without control they become obese. The combination of the attractive food and titbits with no need to hunt for food (exercise), leads very quickly to obesity. This matches human behaviour.

Wherever we look today—supermarkets, service stations, cafes, corner shops, hospital corridors, post offices, etc.—food is readily and easily accessed. Most are low fibre concentrates of sugar and/or fat, often with a high dose of salt. Furthermore, most contain rapid-release carbohydrates, which give us only a temporary energy boost and also give very little in the way of nutrients.

Did you know that appetite and hunger are the result of the body being told that it needs more nutrients—vitamins, minerals, protein, and so on? It is not because the stomach is empty. A person can graze all day on crisps, pizzas, pies, sandwiches, and fizzy drinks but never satisfy the feeling of hunger because those foods do not contain enough of what the body craves: nutrients. A slim vegetarian almost never suffers from hunger!

Not only are these foods attractively packaged, but they also appeal to our taste buds and sense of smell. They play an important role in promoting obesity. If we eat a diet based mainly on sandwiches, pies, sweets, crisps, chocolates, pizzas, pasties, kebabs, burgers, wraps, chips, and so on, it is very hard to satisfy our hunger without overeating.

These foods fail to give us permanent energy. Almost all our energy comes from carbohydrates. Most carbohydrates come from wheat, potatoes, and sugar. All carbohydrates eventually turn into sugar or glucose. Sugar is our energy source, and we need lots of it. But it needs to come with a proper balance of nutrients, and it needs to come from slow-release carbohydrates, as explained earlier.

Foods high in sugar and salt are also habit forming. Processed carbohydrates give us instant sugar boosts and equally instant troughs in energy, making us feel that we need more energy.

How does this happen? When our blood receives glucose there is an instant demand for insulin, which comes from glands in our pancreas. Without insulin, the glucose cannot be absorbed into the cells. If there is a rush of glucose from a chocolate bar, there must also be a rush of insulin to prevent too much glucose being present in the blood, which could lead to a fit. So the glucose is absorbed rapidly. But it leaves the blood drained of glucose, and this is equivalent to feeling tired. You experience a drop in energy.

Naturally, we look for a pick-me-up. More glucose, please! We reach for a cup of coffee, an energy bar, a bun, crisps, a sandwich, a wrap, a biscuit—almost anything that we see nearby. But we remain constantly hungry. Unless we eat the right balance of slow-release carbohydrates and nutrients, we will feel hungry.

We have trillions of cells in our body. In order to work properly they must be slightly alkaline. If they become too acidic, they stop producing enough energy. Every single cell produces a tiny amount of energy called ATP. In addition, each cell has a little pump called a sodium pump, which is meant to keep levels of acidity in check. If the pump does not get sufficient energy, it fails to work properly, and the cell can become too acidic. When this happens, the output of energy declines. Multiply this by trillions, and the result is a tired person.

Processed food makes our cells more acidic. Protein such as meat, fish, milk, cheese and eggs contains acid, meaning that it can lead to higher levels of acid in the cells. Vegetables contain potassium, which is alkaline, and is required for the cells to function properly and produce optimim levels of energy.

The foods which are most acid-forming are refined sugars and processed foods, such as bread and pasta, and almost all food found in a packet, jar, or tin due often to the enormous amount of salt found in these foods. Junk food is very acid-forming. Proteins such as meat are also acidic as are coffee, alcohol and tea.

The answer is simple. The more vegetables you eat, the more energy you will manufacture. But you still need slow-release carbohydrates like oats and brown rice.

Chapter Three

Where did it all start?

Coupled with the availability and marketing of fat-making foods and drinks, our society has become less physically active. The majority of people do not participate in any form of exercise, nor do they go to the shops on foot. Increasingly we are shopping on line which means even less exercise. Most people do not need as much energy as they did years ago because they now have so many mod cons, such as washing machines, cars, electric lawn mowers, dishwashers, computers etc. We are all more sedentary, so we burn fewer calories—but we eat more processed foods than ever. A fine recipe for weight gain and a feeling of listlessness! But even slim people often feel tired because, although they do not eat so much food or may have a more rapid metabolism, they are eating processed foods which do not contain slow-release energy or enough nutrients to stem the feeling of hunger. A person eating a sensible diet will have enough energy to cope and will also be slim.

In 1991, a national food survey showed that the average calorie intake had in fact declined, but physical activity had declined even more. Today, we are less active than in 1991, but we have started to eat more calories because the processed food market has become more powerful. We now see 'healthy' fruit drinks which have over 600 calories per litre made up from sucrose, the sugar from fruit. These drinks are very far from healthy.

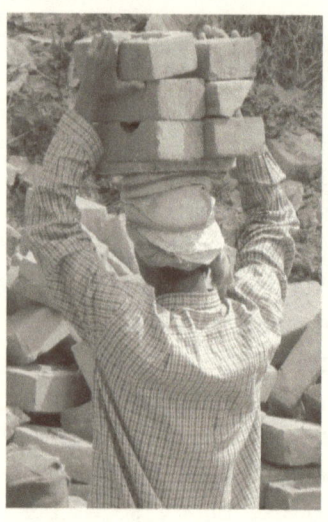 People used to work in industries like mining, steel manufacture, and shipbuilding, and women performed labour intensive housework. In these areas, human muscle has now been replaced by the power of machines. In those days, not only were there less fat people due to the amount of calories being burnt, but there was far less processed food available. Most food was fresh and went mouldy if not eaten shortly after purchase. Most people in manual work needed an enormous amount of energy, so their diets needed to contain lots of carbohydrates, such as potatoes, suet, pastry, pies, and pasties. This was essential fuel, but

at the same time, most families ate vegetables because they were cheap and traditional. They also ate fruit if they could afford it. It did not matter so much that the carbohydrates were rapid-release because they burnt off the calories relatively quickly. Some marathon runners today will eat masses of pasta the night before the event and there don't appear to be many fat marathon runners!!.

Just look at the statistics:

From 1979-1989, energy consumption per person per day fell from 1,750 calories to 1,500, a drop of 14 per cent. For males aged 18-34, energy consumption dropped from 2,500 calories to 1,950, a drop of 22 per cent. No one knows what the figures would show today (2013), but I am sure you would agree that energy consumption will have risen whilst energy expenditure will have dropped.

Today it is important to consume less food, but food with higher nutrient values, and to accept that the creeping inactivity affecting most individuals has reduced our true physiological energy requirement down to a level that fails to satisfy our desire to eat. In other words, we desire to eat more calories than we need because we are not active enough. It is a major dilemma for automated societies. Chapter 11 explains why we eat even if we are not hungry.

Research shows that in 1949 the daily requirement of calories for males aged 18-34 was a colossal 3,400. In 1969 this had fallen to 2,900 calories, and in 1989 to

1,750 calories, so that in just forty years the requirement had halved. Assuming that the pattern continues, by 2029 the daily requirement could be as low as 900 calories, but today most men in that category consume about 2,000 calories. It is easy to see where the problem lies: decreasing activity and too many calories lead to obesity and its associated fatigue.

Chapter Four

Fatigue and obesity— what does it mean?

Put simply, it means an increase in weight and an increase in fat caused by eating the wrong type of carbohydrates and burning fewer calories than consumed. This condition is detrimental to health and well-being. Its effects include restriction of movement and exercise, poor self-image, and social difficulties, as well as countless health disadvantages. Most importantly, it means a fatigue which always leads to irritation, depression, sluggishness, and low self-esteem.

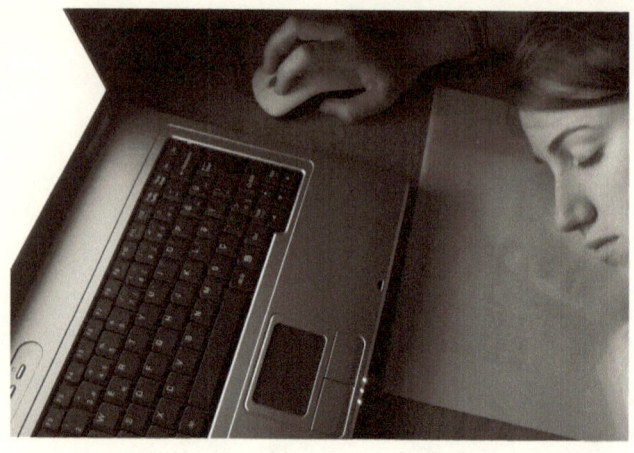

How do we measure obesity?

There are many variables. In the modern world, there has been great intermixing of ethnic and racial groups, resulting in wide genetic variations, such as height, body circumference, and skeletal structure, which complicates the question of how to classify normal weight.

The insurance industry has come up with a formula which includes height, frame size, age, and health. This is probably the best available measure, but it only works for middle-class people who can afford the insurance.

This measure also assumes that whatever weight is desirable at age 21 is also desirable at 45 or 65, but most people increase in weight from ages 20-60, with a gradual decline into old age.

Professor J. S. Garrow, an obesity specialist, came up with a simple measure called the Body Mass Index

(BMI), a ratio of weight to height. If you want to know if you are officially obese, you must measure yourself using the following chart.

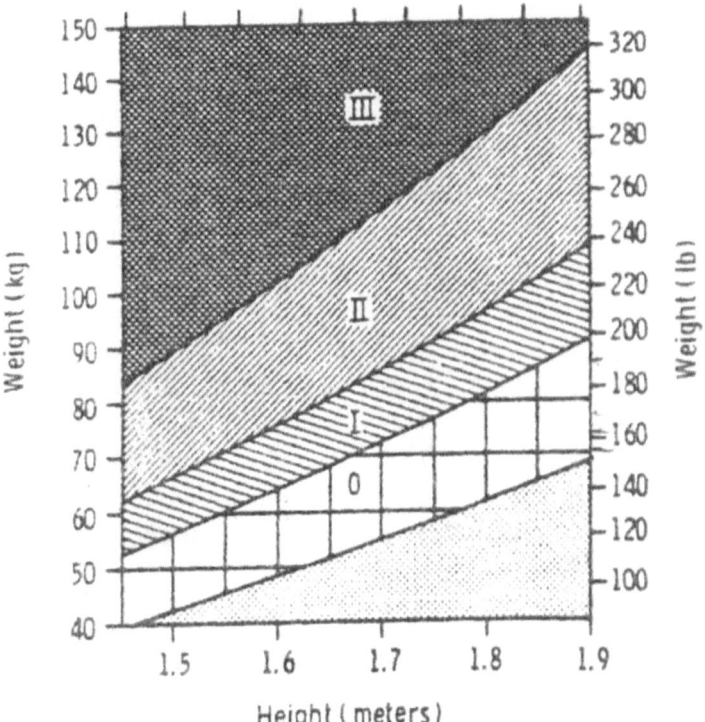

The chart will tell you whether you are overweight and by how much. Regrettably, there are no honest mitigating circumstances. In other words, the chart does not lie.

You should aim to be in the 0 section,.

Insurance companies agree with most of the results from this measurement because they are able to predict how likely you are to die prematurely. There is irrefutable evidence that obesity leads not only to ill health but to premature death.

Obesity and children

Studies have shown that, across the Western world, over one-third of infants are too heavy, and that obesity begins with infancy. Do you have a baby or a young child?

In the USA, over 50 per cent of infants, children, and teenagers are overweight. The figures in the UK and Europe are catching up with the USA. It is a desperately sad situation causing untold misery, but it is so commonplace that the alarm bells have stopped ringing.

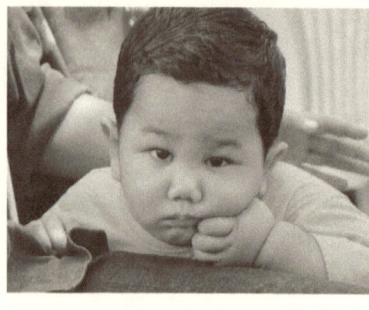

If you have children, ask yourself if they have boundless energy or too much energy or not enough energy or do they have peaks and troughs of energy?. Are they slim, happy, and forever into physical activity? They, more than ever, need slow-release carbohydrates with plenty of nutrients for a growing body. If they are listless, always tired, and overweight, perhaps you should examine their diet. If they are over active, perhaps you should examine their diet. Are you a mum or dad who allows your children to eat sweets and treats whenever you think they have done well, or you just want them to be quiet? Do you know how much this will lead to problems for them in the future? Do you allow your child to waste food? Would that be because they demand more than they can eat, or is it because they know that they can snack on junk food in between meals?

Do your children have boundless energy and therefore sleep like a log at night? Or do they sit up all night in front of a computer or phone, munching on crisps, waking up late and listless? Do they then give you a hard time all day because they are tired and drained of energy? Or do they scream and shout whenever they want something? Is your child overactive? Is the problem made worse because you too are tired and drained?

Try changing your diet and theirs too. Children need 3 meals daily with plenty of slow release carbohydrates in the morning and at lunch but much less in the evening. They also need masses of exercise. They need vegetables and a little fruit and should avoid processed or junk food and fizzy drinks. Crisps and sweets are just fuelling disaster. Feed your child properly and you will be amazed at the difference in their behaviour.

Chapter Five

The risks of early death

Cardiovascular diseases

These diseases are aggravated by high blood pressure, increased fat in the blood, and increased sugar levels, which all occur with obesity. For every 10 per cent rise in weight, blood pressure increases by 6.5 mm, cholesterol increases by 12 mg, and sugar increases by 2 mg. Any increase in weight into grades 1, 2, or 3 on the BMI scale will increase the risks associated with blood pressure, sugar levels, and cholesterol levels, all of which may increase the risk of early death.

Diabetes

It is a well known fact that obesity and type 2 diabetes are firm bedfellows, and diabetes is not much fun. Once again, the fatter the individual, the higher the chances of diabetes. The connection between diabetes and rapid-release carbohydrates is evident. Fatigue is also a bedfellow of, and a precursor to, diabetes for the reasons given above.

Hypertension/stress

When a person's weight increases, their blood pressure will rise accordingly. Therefore, weight loss will trigger a similar lowering of blood pressure. The three factors affecting this are sodium/salt content, nervousness, and hormone imbalance, all of which play a part in your levels of blood pressure.

Breathing

As a person gets fatter, so the muscular work required for breathing increases. If the lungs don't function fully, retention of carbon dioxide occurs, which leads to lethargy and sleepiness. In chronic (long-term) cases of obesity, a higher than normal red blood cell count may develop, which may increase the risk of thrombosis, respiratory disease, hypertension in the lungs, heart enlargement, and congestive heart failure.

Gall bladder disease

Increased body fat is associated with increased cholesterol production, so it is easier for cholesterol stones to form.

Arthritis

The more weight being carried, the greater the wear and tear on the joints, leading sometimes to osteoarthritis.

Gout

Uric acid is often the culprit in gout. Obese people have more uric acid, so the heavier you are, the more likely you are to suffer from this painful condition.

Breast and endometrial cancer

The endometrium is the lining of the womb. A greater risk of breast and womb cancer may occur in obese women due to endocrine or hormone abnormalities and an increased conversion of one oestrogen to another in fatty tissues. This is a little complicated to understand, but research indicates a connection between obesity and cancer of the breast and womb lining.

Genetics

Many studies have shown that there is a genetic link between fat parents and fat children. It is also true that children grow fatter as their parents grow fatter. This is not surprising since the diet fat parents eat will be given to their children. Professor Garrow has suggested from a wide range of findings that more than 25 per cent of the factors tending towards obesity are of genetic origin. It would follow that if parents care about their children, they will ensure that the children do not become obese, by following a better diet themselves.

Hormones

Many people believe that an imbalance in their endocrine system is the cause of their obesity, but this disorder is rarely the cause. The opposite is much more likely. Obesity can, and often does, cause an imbalance to the endocrine system. This leads to an increase in growth hormone, cortisol, and insulin, which can have negative effects.

Chapter Six

Slimming diets and thermogenesis

Put really simply thermogenesis means that if an overwieght person eats the same calories as a slim person, more of the calories consumed by that person will be available as extra energy deposited as fat. This means that fewer calories are required because so many calories are already stored as fat.

Some scientists do not believe that this has much impact upon obesity, usually because they work for companies with a vested interest in selling slimming products. Studies on rats, however, conclude that fat rats are more disposed to being fat, even if on exactly the same diet as thin ones. This means that they either exercise less or have a slower metabolism (burn energy more slowly). Either there is a gene (or genes) that favours or discourages thermogenesis, or some rats are just lazier than others.

Energy expenditure

The using up of energy takes three forms: basal metabolic rate (BMR), physical activity, and the thermic effect of food.

BMR is the amount of energy required to maintain the trillions of cells in the body. Children have a high BMR because so much energy is required for growing. Obese people have a higher BMR than slim people because they need more energy to move about because they are heavier. However, their BMR is lower than that of slim people when measured as a per kilo of body weight, explaining why obese people feel so tired.

Ten per cent of all our energy is used up in digestion. This leads to a reduction in the production of heat by about the same percentage, so eating causes a drop in our body temperature. Insulin may be required for this effect, so obese people may depend upon their insulin sensitivity for the necessary production of digestive energy. Since insulin balance is sometimes threatened in obese people, this can become a problem.

Weight gain and energy expenditure

A study of children showed that the total energy expenditure measured at three months, was 20.7 per cent lower in infants who at one year of age, had become overweight, than it was in infants who had not, suggesting that decreased energy expenditure might lead to weight gain.

Is exercise good for us?

A very recent study from a leading London university makes it quite clear that the reduction of activity in young children has led to the increase in chronic illnesses. It seems to make no difference how many studies are done offering the same information, nobody in government is willing to do anything about it except ask for yet another study. Obesity causes miserable side effects and ultimately leads to years of suffering and ill health before premature death, while costing our health service vast sums of tax payers' money. Chronic fatigue has also reached epidemic proportions, but because it is so common and is not seen as a disorder. It is taken for granted, though it also leads to a difficult life full of stresses and strains that often have a dreadful impact upon family life.

Fat cells

This section is bad news for obese people. As explained earlier, fat cells can expand to contain more fat, and they can multiply. When a fat cell is full, a new one is created. This potential increase in fat cell numbers has no bounds. The bad news is that the number of fat cells doesn't appear to decrease when weight is lost.

In becoming obese, you have manufactured additional fat cells, and they will never go away. It is much easier to fill a large number of fat cells just a little bit than it is to fill a small amount of fat cells a lot. That is why it is so difficult to lose weight.

When you are overweight, you have to reduce the amount of fat in many more cells than when you were slim, and then you have to avoid consuming fat-making foods because the fat is so easily stored in the increased number of fat cells. It is easier to lose the fat from five cells than from ten, but it is easier to store fat in ten cells than in five. Obese people are in a lose/lose situation.

Dietary management

No one needs to be told that losing weight and keeping it off is extremely difficult, particularly for those who are 25 per cent or more overweight. But some knowledge of nutrition can help.

Protein

Fat, carbohydrates, and protein all contribute reasonably equivalently, calorie for calorie, to diet-induced thermogenesis (the production of heat), resulting in equal calories available for fat deposit. In other words, high protein diets won't help.

Impaired absorption

Dietary fibre, non-digestible fat substitutes, starch blockers, and other agents have all been suggested as absorption inhibitors. Their success has not only been limited but can cause nasty side effects due to fat and carbohydrate malabsorption.

Fasts

The problem with total fasts is that it is not just fat that is lost. Everything is lost, and it is hard to replace. Mineral and other micronutrient loss is also evident.

Protein-supplemented modified fasts have increased in popularity. These produce 400-700 calories that generate rapid weight loss. The protein comes as a shake, supplement, or as lean meat, fowl, or fish. It is dangerous to use these diets for longer than sixteen weeks, although clients can lose 1.5 to 2.3 kilos per week on these diets. The protein needs to be of high biologic quality to prevent the loss of our own body protein. Many of the health benefits of a good diet are sacrificed in order to lose weight quickly, but at a cost to your health. Once the diet is over, what then? The folks supplying you with these quick-fix diets want you to come back after you have put the weight back on. I know a number of people who use these diets for special occasions like weddings and holidays. They lose weight quickly and then pile it back on until the next occasion. This is a great strategy for someone's profits.

Ketogenic diets

There are a variety of diets based upon gluconeogenesis, something Mr Atkins knew about. In these diets, carbohydrates make up less than 20 per cent of the diet, so they cease to be an adequate source of energy. As a generalisation, there is a high intake of protein which is converted into energy through a process called gluconeogenesis. Because the body is denied the correct

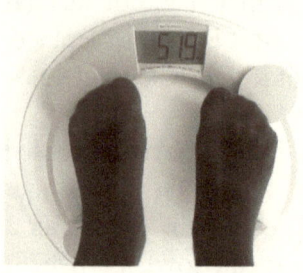 amount of carbohydrates, greater amounts of energy are needed to convert protein into energy. Since the main source of energy (carbohydrates) has been reduced, and more energy is required to convert

protein into energy, it means that energy stored in the fat cells is used up rapidly.

The danger is that since the body only requires small amounts of protein, any excess is converted into ammonia and then into uric acid (think gout), putting undue pressure on our kidneys and risking toxic side effects, such as nausea, hypertension, fatigue, aches, pains, and bad breath.

Most of these diets are low in fibre due to their near absence of fruit and vegetables, which can lead to constipation. Furthermore, valuable vitamins and minerals may be missing. Over a short period, they do work should you wish to risk it and spend a lot of money.

Of the patients who lose significant amounts of weight, 80-100 per cent will regain it.

A person reducing weight requires less energy, unless exercising, and this causes a drop of about 15-30 per cent of metabolic rate, the rate at which energy is used. It becomes more difficult to lose weight on the <u>same</u> diet in the second month than the first, and more difficult in the third than the second, and so on. A person losing weight rapidly will almost certainly regain weight within three months, so where's the point? The point is very simple: it may have taken more than five years to become obese, so it may take five years to become slim again.

Studies show that obese people who have lost weight have a lowered calorie requirement which may persist for years. If daily calorie intake is increased above one thousand per day, weight gain will occur. When trying to lose weight, you must decrease the calories you consume a little more each month until you reach the weight you require. Unless you take exercise, you have to continue to consume less than one thousand calories daily, which is very hard to do.

Once you have been overweight, you will require fewer calories than a lean or slim person, even years after having lost the weight, which seems so very unfair. Some major slimming outfits that use a points system, but fail to tell their paying clients that, as each month passes, their bodies need less food. Their points system should reflect that fact. That is the way the body responds to having been overweight. Tough, but true.

The answer

In view of the risks involved in extreme, slimming and protein based diets and the prolonged periods of time that restricted diets must be followed, a well-balanced mixed diet is the only sensible approach to weight loss.

Diets in the 1,100-1,200 calorie range can include appropriate macro- and micronutrients, vitamins, and proteins. They can be followed for months without supplements but are safer with supplements. The supplements generally required are zinc, folic acid, and vitamin B6.

Protein should be raised to about sixty grams daily, giving about 260 calories which will constitute 25 per cent of total calories.

Slow release carbohydrates will constitute 30 per cent and fat 20 per cent of the total diet, the remainder coming from fibre. in the form of fruit and vegetables.

Fat-soluble vitamins and essential fatty acids will be available from fat and fibre and anti-ketogenic (energy from protein) effects will come from carbohydrates.

Following a diet of this kind needs professional advice, but your energy levels will increase greatly, and the increase will be permanent because you will consume the correct balance of nutrients. But I repeat that it is essential to speak to a properly qualified nutritionist before embarking on this sort of diet.

Chapter Seven

The alternatives

Before taking exercise

It is nonsense to tell people to take exercise if they are feeling exhausted. The best step to take is to change your diet for a month, which should give you more energy, before you try to take exercise. During the first month you will begin to feel a little more energy creeping into you, and with some luck you will also begin to sleep better. Persevere with your new diet, and during the second month, you may feel more like beginning to take some exercise.

Exercise

If you can take exercise, so much the better. This is not rocket science. If you burn up more calories than you consume, you will lose weight. Exercise helps to burn calories, though you must remember that calorie charts can be misleading.

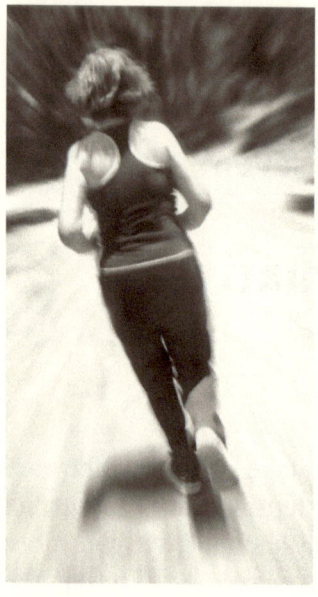

Take this example: An obese person exercising on a treadmill at 4 mph would burn off 210 calories over thirty minutes, but 39 calories would have been burnt off by sitting in a chair over the same time. The 39 calories have to be deducted from the 210 in order to realise the real benefit of the treadmill exercise: 171 calories.

Some say that exercise inhibits eating, but there is no evidence of this. In lean or slim people, exercise encourages them to restock their calorie loss, so be warned: exercise might make you feel hungry. Then there is the reward factor. Having exercised, it is easy to feel that a reward is deserved. You may find yourself eating a high calorie treat after exercise.

Exercise will help attain weight loss while allowing less difficult diets to be consumed.

The truth is that if you want to enjoy your food intake, exercise will probably be required in some form or another.

Drugs

Drugs are used in some cases by doctors, but the side effects can be disastrous. Appetite suppressants are used to induce anorexia, and many are amphetamines. They are seldom used without the support of a transformative diet and exercise.

Psychotherapy

There is not a lot of weight loss success reported in this field. All sorts of people are fat, and most do not have a psychological problem, unless you count overeating and being under active as a psychological problem.

Behaviour modification

Huge amounts of literature have been written on this subject. Modification programmes include keeping diaries: records of what and when was eaten, where, with whom, how (sitting, standing, walking), emotions, and frequency of hunger. Food management, such as buying, storing, preparing, serving, and cleaning of food is also recorded. Techniques include eating more slowly, smaller amounts, smaller plates, rewards, where and with whom you eat and so on. Very little success appears to have been recorded using these techniques, but some people may value them.

Surgical treatment

Surgical treatments include a shortening of the bowel to reduce absorption of food, a reduction in stomach size to reduce calorie intake, and jaw wiring for 6-9 months to prevent large quantities of food from being eaten.

All of these treatments are radical, but are used when obesity becomes life threatening. More recently, an inflatable balloon device can be inserted into the stomach which makes eating large quantities impossible.

It would appear that most alternative treatments for obesity fail.

Chapter Eight

The answers to fatigue

Recognise that you are overtired and overweight and challenged.

Recognise that you were not always like this, and that you can return to your desired weight.

Never ever make another excuse for your condition. Excuses are props and will hold you back from tackling the problem.

Don't aim too high. Give yourself years rather than months to reach your goal.

Accept that there are no magic wands, and that only your effort and determination will get you there.

Accept the simplicity and accept the changes. Never say, 'I can't.' Instead say, 'I can, I will,' and smile while you say it even though you may be gritting your teeth.

What do I do to find lost energy and lose weight?

It's all contained in what you eat. I see increasing numbers of weary and fat people of all ages: children, babies, grannies, granddads, mums, dads, and single men and women. I often see them walking in the streets eating crisps, sweets, pasties, pies, sandwiches, and so on. These people graze all day because they are tired and hungry and often depressed, and no matter how much they eat, they remain tired and hungry.

Hunger is triggered by the body's requirement for nutrients: vitamins, minerals, and phytonutrients. The foods which people graze or snack on do not satisfy appetite. The carbohydrates found in fast foods, snacks, and fizzy drinks give a short-lived energy shot which rapidly gives way to a drop in energy levels and a sense of fatigue. This fatigue is translated into a demand for more energy. Since the person suffering from fatigue only ever eats rapid-release carbohydrates in the form of crisps, sandwiches, wraps, pies, cakes, muffins, sweets, and chocolates, all washed down with a fizzy drink or coffee, the body simply gets another shot of energy and never enough of the nutrients which would stem the urge for more food. This vicious cycle inevitably leads to weight gain and fatigue.

What's the excuse?

Wherever we look—supermarkets, service stations, corner shops, schools, hospital canteens, almost everywhere we can buy food—we are faced with a barrage of sweets, crisps, pies, sandwiches, muffins, cakes, and masses of sugar-filled canned and bottled drinks.

The first thing you must do is to avoid buying any of these products, which from now on will be known as processed food: the enemy.

A processed food diet for a day

	Protein	Fats	Carbs/Sugar	Fibre	Calories
Breakfast					
Cereal	2	0.2	34	0.4	136
Milk	2.6	3.2	4	0	54
Snack					
Biscuits	2.3	11	28	1	214
Coke	0	0	15	0	57
Lunch					
Baked Beans	7.3	1	21	9	118
Chips	4	5	36	3	195
Pie	14	33	40	1.6	506
Ketchup	0.3	0	3.4	0	14
Coke	0	0	15	0	57
Snack					
Lemonade	0	0	10	0	39
Dinner					
Chicken Soup	2.5	6	7	0	86
Peas	6	1	15	0	86
Mashed Potatoes	2	0	18	4	75
Burgers	21	5.5	1.3	0	272
White Bread	9	1	61	3	277
Butter	0	10	0	0	87
Totals	68	92	313	24	2776
	13.6%	18.4%	62.6%	4.8%	

A balanced diet

	Protein	Fats	Carbs/Sugar	Fibre	Calories
	12%	12%	50%	26%	1800

This processed food diet contains 13 per cent too much carbohydrate, and it is all rapid-release carbohydrate, leading to peaks and troughs in energy levels.

There is too little fibre, leading to constipation, bloating, IBS, and possible bowel cancer.

Fats and oils are too high, adding unwanted calories.

The amount of protein is not bad, but it is not varied enough.

In short, this diet will lead to obesity, a loss of energy, and chronic ill health if continued over a lifetime.

If you read on, you will begin to understand how empty the processed diet really is, and why it leads to fatigue and hunger.

Minerals are extremely important because without them the body cannot convert food into all the chemicals required for proper functioning. We need a wide range: sodium/salt, calcium, potassium, phosphorous, zinc, magnesium, iron, copper, and manganese are the main ones. In order to keep things simple, we will look at sodium, calcium, and potassium, and lump all the others together even though each one has an important part to play.

Do you remember what acidosis is? Our body should be mildly alkaline because we were designed to be alkaline. If we become more acidic than alkaline, our body stops functioning normally. The first sign of that is fatigue.

Every cell in the body produces a tiny amount of energy. Every cell also contains a sodium pump which pumps out acid and keeps the cell topped up with potassium, which keeps the cell from becoming acidic. If there is a drop in energy output, the sodium pump will not function effectively, allowing the cell to become acidic. This, in turn, reduces the amount of energy the cell produces, and so the process spirals downhill, leading eventually to chronic disorders and a malfunctioning cell, or even a diseased cell. The first sign of this is fatigue.

In order to remain slightly alkaline, we must eat food with lots of potassium and some calcium, and we must not eat food containing lots of salt/sodium. If we eat too much protein, we will become more acidic because most animal food (a source of protein) is acid forming. Your food should contain much more potassium than sodium/salt. Calcium is also alkaline-forming, but we should not eat too much of it, so eat less cheese and cow's milk and yogurt.

In the empty diet above, we have, in grams:

Sodium	4220	50%
Potassium	2583	30%
Calcium	550	15%
Remainder	160	5%

Our body requires more potassium than sodium, and the levels of calcium and the remainder are far too low. These levels will produce a highly acid diet which is self destructive. Having acidic cells leads to fatigue and mineral loss and eventually chronic illness.

Now for the vitamins. Most of the diet gives us a deficiency of vitamins. Coke, lemonade, and processed peas produce nothing of value. Vitamins A and D are found in milk and butter; Vitamins B3, B4, and B5 are found in items like chips, cereal, and burgers; B6 and B12 are found in the pie and the burger; and folate is found in the cereal, beans, chips, and the soup. Vitamin C is found in the chips and is almost absent elsewhere. Overall, vitamins are not in plentiful supply in this diet.

Contrast

In order to make the point, I have chosen a super diet which is extreme but demonstrates the contrast, in a somewhat exaggerated way. Your super diet can be eaten throughout the day and is made up as follows.

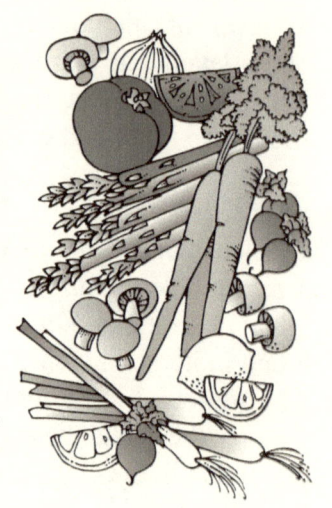

Consider that the values come from a large portion of each of the items of food.

	Pro-tein	Fat	Sug-ar	Fi-bre	Salt	Potas-sium	Cal-cium	Re-mainder	Vitamins	Calo-ries
Cabbage	7	1.6	16	12	20	1080	217	200	Good	104
Cucumber	1	0.1	6	3	9	200	34	76	Good	13
Courgette	1.8	0.4	1.6	1.7	1	390	34	68	Very good	18
Broccoli	36	7	15	0	70	3200	465	980	Excellent	300
Lettuce	0.6	0.4	0.8	0.8	3	240	39	35	Excellent	8
Chicory	0.4	0.4	2.3	0	1	165	26	33	Fair	9
Turnips	7	3.5	39	31	126	2333	400	410	Fair	191
Radish	0.3	0	0.9	0.4	3	200	25	180	Fair	9
Brussels Sprouts	3	1	3	2.5	3	250	17	57	Very good	30
Brown Rice	10	4	122	5	4	375	15	639	Fair	639
Millet	11	3	75	0	6	505	23	505	Poor	380

This slightly unrealistic diet offers:

Carbohydrates	55%
Protein	16%
Fibre	18%
Fats/Oils	11%
Calories	1590
Salt	4%
Potassium	28%
Calcium	20%
Remainder	48%

A balanced diet is much more realistic than a super diet, but what this shows is that good food must contain plenty of vitamins, minerals, and plenty of fibre. It must have more potassium than sodium so that the body is more alkaline than acid, and 50 per cent must be energy food—better known as slow-releasing carbohydrates.

Chapter Nine

Your energy-gain diet— month one

You need a balanced diet of slow-release carbohydrates for your energy levels. It is better to eat these in the morning at breakfast and at lunch time. Slow-release carbohydrates include oats, brown rice and millet. You must have enough energy in the morning, or you will start to snack because you feel tired.

Breakfast

Homemade muesli every morning of the week.

Recipe

Make enough for a month at a time.
1 kilo of organic oats
150 grams of oat bran
150 grams of wheat bran
150 grams of psyllium powder
100 grams of mixed nuts
100 grams of mixed seeds
50 grams of raisins
50 grams of sultanas
50 grams of linseeds

Some of these items are readily available but some can be bought in a health food shop.

Mix thoroughly into a large plastic tub. When poured into a bowl, add one or more of the following: blueberries, blackberries, strawberries, apricots, or prunes.

Add either, soya, goat, oat, or rice milk. If there are things in this mixture you do not like, don't add them. If there are other things you like similar to these things, add them. You must like what you eat, but do try really hard not to add cow's milk because it will upset the calcium levels in your diet.

Lunch

You are about to become a soup magician. You will make and consume three to four litres of home-made vegetable soups each week to eat at lunch times and/or in the evenings. If you are not at home for lunch, take it to work in a flask.

Go to the recipe page at www.riverford.co.uk and look up soups to gain some useful tips on how vegetable soups can be really exciting and full of flavour. Do not make only well-known soups, such as carrot and coriander or tomato and basil. These are just so boring. Be adventurous, and invent new soups without names. Be imaginative and creative: use any and all vegetables—don't be afraid to use four or more at a time.

Raw and cooked vegetables can cause a lot of wind, so use a blender until your tummy settles down and you get used to them. Try not to use cubes for thickeners—they contain masses of salt. Use onions, leeks, stock from last night's meal, lentils, or sweet potatoes to thicken soups. Use herbs and spices, mustard, or lemon—anything to give your soups that 'wow' factor. Some soups won't come off so well. Don't despair, add something like tomatoes to change the taste.

Don't waste your food. If you have leftovers from dinner, chuck them into your soup.

Always remain hygienic with your soups. Never keep them for too long, and always wash up properly.

If you have a friend who is also trying to lose weight, compare notes on soups. Experiment together—it's much more fun. If you become good enough, write a recipe book and publish it as an e-book.

Enjoy your soups. They are so low in calories and so nutritious and full of fibre.

Dinner

If you feel exhausted, get home late, or just cannot be bothered, have soup with a salad, or an avocado pear and trout fillet on some rye bread—something light and quick.

Otherwise, you can eat fish or meat or fowl and vegetables, but no puddings. For filling food at dinner time, try brown rice or millet or a little sweet potato or savoury potato. Brown rice needs to be cooked for forty minutes, and millet is best steamed. Potatoes are OK, but you will take longer to lose weight if you eat potatoes, as they contain a lot of starch. Begin to serve yourself less meat and potatoes until small portions of meat are satisfying. Eat as much fish as you like and do not be afraid of eating eggs. Stir fries are a good option too. Have more vegetables at dinner. If you have a sluggish digestive system, you should try eating more vegetables so as to raise your levels of fibre.

Oats is your core morning carbohydrate, your energy source. Soups are your lunch, containing wonderful fibre and all the vitamins and minerals you need. Your soups will contain carbohydrates if you thicken them with beans, root vegetables, or potatoes, but you need energy and will burn it off if you become physically active. Try walking a little more or get a bike. But be warned that carbohydrates eaten at night/dinner time tend to add to your weight because you do not normally burn them off unless you're very active at night. Have only small portions of brown rice, millet or potatoes at night.

Limit fruit to a maximum of two pieces daily because of their sugar content. I suggest one portion with your muesli, and a banana as a snack.

What to avoid

In the first month you absolutely must avoid all traces of wheat. No bread, pasta, pies, pasties, pastries, rolls, cakes, biscuits, wraps, couscous, or anything made from processed wheat. No processed or white rice either.

This is imperative

No cow dairy produce—no cow's milk, yogurt, or cheese. You can use goat, soya, sheep, oat, or rice milk products but no cheeses. This is for the first month only. Do not put milk in your coffee or tea. Have you ever tried redbush or rooibosch tea with a bit of honey and lemon juice? It's a wonderful drink full of antioxidants and has no caffeine.

Cow's milk contains casein, which is the protein in milk, and it is hard to digest. It also contains lactose, which is the name for the sugar in milk. It also contains high levels of salt, so steer clear of milk for a month. Be warned! A cup of coffee contains about 6 calories. Large milky coffees can contain up to 350 calories or more.

Finally, absolutely no processed food at all

Avoiding processed food is difficult because it is around us all the time. This rule means no pies, pasties, bread, rolls, biscuits, cakes, crisps, chips, sweets, chocolates, and almost anything that is in a can, a glass container, a package, or a tube.

Go to your fridge or food store and look for some whole, natural fresh food. Most of what you can see will be in a packet, bottle, can, or wrapper of some sort. From now on you will have to prepare your food and use the microwave oven less often.

Food is processed for a number of reasons, storage, transport and profit. Fresh food contains bacteria. Human beings need natural bacteria to help our own bacteria which lives in our gut, so that the two sources of bacteria help to digest our food. Processed food has diminished levels of bacteria.

Processing destroys the bacteria. Processed food also spends longer in the gut because the absence of fibre causes bloating and constipation. Not only does processed food require more bacteria to aid its digestion, but it provides less bacteria. It is a lose-lose situation.

Fresh food has more of the bacteria which aids digestion. Fresh food becomes mouldy more rapidly because its own bacteria digests it. But we need this process to occur in our gut to aid digestion.

Processed food may remain on the shelves, in our fridges, in supermarket cabinets, in cans, etc., for weeks. This is after it has been transported around the world. Not only does modern food last for ages without going mouldy, but it is packaged to appear inviting and tempting. It usually smells good when heated up because of added flavours, and it appears so attractive because of added colourings.

Disappointingly, we have to accept the destruction of the food. Processing denudes the food of many of its minerals and vitamins. The more it is processed, the less value it contains.

We pay a lot of money for a product which is of less nutritional value, has almost no fibre, is usually laced with salt and or sugar, but has wonderful flavour, wonderful appearance, and is easy to prepare.

I never stop asking myself why people are prepared to waste their money on this stuff. It is of less nutritional value and costs more per gram of nutrients than fresh food. Don't eat any processed foods during the first month.

If you manage to do this without snacking or taking shortcuts, you should manage to consume less than one thousand two hundred calories daily but have more energy than before.

Chapter Ten

Your energy-gain diet— month two

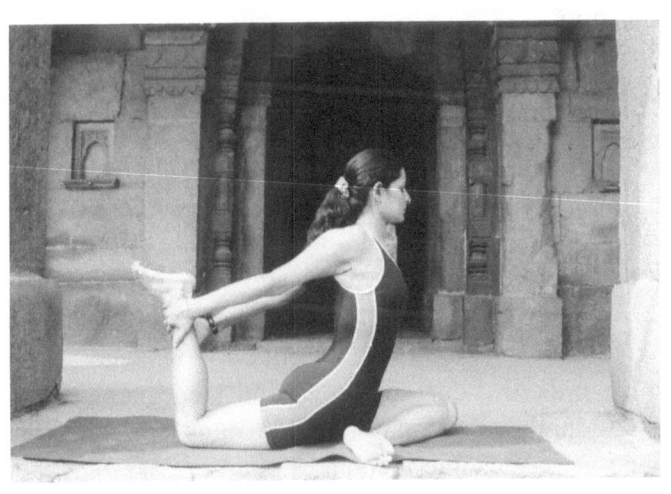

Assuming you get this far, you can take your foot off the pedal a little. You should have more energy, and you should be feeling better as well as having lost a little weight. You should be going to the toilet properly on a daily basis. If not, your digestion is not functioning as it should, and you will struggle to lose any weight at all.

If your digestive system is sluggish, you must eat a lot of fibre. The vegetable soups should help, as should the psyllium powder, oat bran, and wheat bran in your muesli. If you are desperate, buy some Epsom salts and take a heaped teaspoon in the evenings. Use a small amount of hot water to dissolve the salts and gulp it in one. It tastes awful, so have some grapes handy. Use the amount of salts required for a regular daily elimination, but for no longer than a month. If you continue to have difficulties, visit your nearest colonic hydrotherapist. Look for a practitioner on the internet but ensure that your practitioner is also qualified in nutrition.

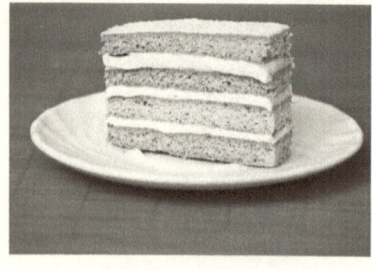 At this point, you may begin moving towards an 80/20 diet. You will eat 80 per cent as you did for the first month and 20 per cent of almost anything you like. You may have some milk in your coffee/tea and some goat cheese occasionally. You may include eggs for breakfast once a week, some alcohol, a slice of cake—in fact,

anything that takes your fancy. But remember that the more you consume of these treats, the more sugar you will consume. Sugar means calories. Carbohydrates = sugar = calories = weight, and carbohydrates like pasta and bread often contain wheat, so try to keep this sort of food very much on the back burner.

You must have a reward, so I suggest that you think of taking some exercise if you haven't done so already. Any sort of exercise that takes your fancy and that burns up calories will do, so a gentle walk with the dog is hardly sufficient. Don't fall for the folly of embracing an aerobics class in order to give yourself a walnut cake and a mega-cappuccino, because you may give up the fitness class, but you will not give up the treat.

All of this regime change must be done with both a sense of adventure and a sense of joy. If you are nervous about joining a running club, go with a friend. Everyone can trot, and every running club has a beginners group. The same applies to swimming, cycling, rambling—the list is endless.

If you want to enjoy the naughty-but-nice treats, you have to find a way of burning off those additional calories. Exercise is excellent for your overall health. You will sleep better, sex will be better, you'll glow, and you'll be able to cope better with stress and children.

A patient came to see me who was suffering from a lack of energy, a few extra pounds, a sluggish digestive system (2-3 eliminations a week), and not much enthusiasm for anything apart from Facebook. This condition applies, in my opinion, to 80 per cent of the population of the Western world.

My patient had a colon cleanse, a month of dietary changes, and a second colon treatment. During the second treatment, she told me that she had begun to get up in the mornings early enough to take her son to school after making his breakfast. Additionally, she had begun to invite friends over to her home after a period of five years of hibernation. Finally, she cancelled her Facebook account where she had 1,400 contacts. She had found energy, lost weight, was no longer sluggish, rediscovered her son, and realised that her life had been slipping away pointlessly.

How did she do this? She ate a home-made muesli mix for breakfast, ate home-made vegetable soups for lunch and as a snack, avoided processed foods, and drank more water. She even began a little gentle jogging. She did it and so can you.

The main ingredients to her success were an oats based cereal in the mornings like Muesli with some fruit, vegetable soups daily, a basic evening meal of a meat or fish and vegetables. Moderate consumption of tea and coffee and about a litre of water each day. She avoided as far as possible rapid release carbohydrates such as white bread and she avoided too much dairy produce and salt. She enjoyed very low consumption of sweet things such as cake but ate 3 pieces of fruit daily. She also enjoyed a few treats each day but only if she had been taking a little exercise.

Chapter Eleven

Why is it so easy to get so tired?

There are a number of reasons. Salt and sugar are both habit-forming. Salt is used as a preservative, so it is an essential part of foods that spend time being transported and sitting in storage and then on shelves in a shop. Sugar is also a preservative, so it is used in a wide range of foods for the same reason. Sugar is also our main source of energy, so if we feel tired we tend to turn to sweet things to replenish our lost energy.

Since most of the foods we see in a supermarket have been transported and stored for a while, we must accept that they probably contain high levels of either salt or sugar or both. Part of the storage story includes the destruction of useful bacteria which are needed to assist our own bacteria in the digestion of foods and empty foods give short sharp hints of energy but not satisfying continuous energy. The problem is further aggravated because the preparation and storage of foods requires processes that destroy a high proportion of nutrients, which mean that those foods are not whole. They are what I describe as empty foods.

Take this example:

A portion of wholemeal flour gives 360 calories.

A similar portion of processed flour gives 396 calories

The processed flour contains 9.4 per cent less protein, 57 per cent less fibre, 78 per cent less vitamin E, 65 per cent fewer B vitamins, and an average of 65 per cent less mineral value.

In the case of polished or processed rice, the mineral loss is even greater, reaching a depletion of 93 per cent of copper, and in the case of vitamins, the average loss is more than 60 per cent. You can see how drastically, important nutrients are eroded in the processing of foods.

Before you complain that fresh food is too expensive, consider the following. If a kilo of whole rice costs £2 and a kilo of processed rice costs £1.50, the processed rice is 25 per cent cheaper. But if the processed rice contains over 60 per cent fewer nutrients, it should cost 60 per cent less than the whole rice: 80p. You would be paying 70p too much for your cheaper rice. Now tell me it is too expensive to buy whole food.

Processed food contains far less fibre and will ultimately lead to a sluggish digestive system with all the knock-on effects. Our bodies absolutely must have fibre, vitamins, and minerals. Processed foods on average have 60 per cent less of these ingredients. That is why I call these foods empty, and why I insist that they have far less value than whole foods. Please do not use the 'it's too expensive' excuse, which in most cases is a euphemism for 'I can't be bothered to prepare and cook food.'

Why do we consume all this rubbish? Because it tastes good, smells good, lasts a long time in storage, is easily prepared or heated, and frequently requires no cooking at all. Far too many people have no idea how to cook, and this is nothing short of a disgrace.

Nevertheless, as you have probably experienced, eat enough of it, and you will feel tired, bloated, overweight, and sluggish. You will also have become a victim of the food manufacturing industry that collectively spends billions on marketing and research persuading governments to be relaxed about what is being done to tempt you into consuming ever increasing amounts of their products, and thereby increasing their profits as fast as possible. Tired, fat people are the food industry's greatest success. People who have been tempted to consume far too much of what they produce—junk!

Finally

If you decide to attempt a new regime in order to gain more energy and lose weight, keep telling yourself that you are at war. At war with all the things that made you feel fat and tired and sluggish and fed up. You are also alone. Only you put food into your mouth, so only you can decide to put less in it, and only you can decide what to put in it.

Now you're going to put the right things in your body. No more rubbish. You're going to find more energy, and the newfound energy will help you stay on track. You are going to cleanse your body from years of junk food build-up, and once you have spent four weeks on a sensible diet, you are going to begin taking some exercise which will enable you to have a few treats. You are going to continue this 80/20 regime for the rest of your life. This is not a temporary situation.

In six months time, your friends and family will remark on how changed you are, how much more energy you have, how much less stressed you are, and how much weight you've lost.

Good luck, good eating, good life.

What clients say

'Having visited my doctor and even a consultant without any successful results, I finally turned to an alternative treatment, more in hope than expectation. The result was almost instant, and although the first few days were difficult, I found that the increase in energy made life so much better that I could face almost any new challenges.'
(Paula, Exmouth)

'I retired early after years of hard work, but after a while found that I had become sluggish and overweight. After seeing a colonic hydrotherapist—doctors don't seem to rate them!—I felt so much better, and the nutritional advice was spot on. I have joined a running club and am fitter than ever, so I can indulge myself from time to time. But I still go to my practitioner every six months.'
(Caroline, Teignmouth)

'I spent more time on Facebook than anything else. My son hardly saw me. I never saw anyone much. I felt so tired all the time. I went to see a practitioner because there was nothing a doctor could do for me. Anyway, after a week or so on a different diet I felt so much better I eventually terminated my Facebook contract and am seeing friends now and doing stuff with my son. Life is so much better.'
(Tracey, Torbay)

'After visiting my practitioner and changing my diet, I felt so good, and all my friends told me that I had changed. My hair was shiny, my skin improved, I was always in a good mood, and I had much more energy. It was so simple, but unless you know what to do you can't get there. Never felt better in all my life.'
(Linda, Exeter)

The author

Educated in East Africa, UK, and at Loughborough University, Peter Taylor taught English and Physical Education, managed leisure centres, organised major events, owned shops in France, lived in Kashmir, and owned a health spa in Devon before embarking on a career as an alternative health practitioner.

With a science degree in Nutrition, he is well-qualified to comment on the extraordinary rise in global fatigue and obesity. Since almost nothing is being done to tackle this immense problem, it is incumbent upon him to draw attention to some of the reasons for this rise.

This booklet is designed to inform and to give those who would like to gain energy, take control, and lose weight, the real truth behind the problems associated with fatigue and obesity. In addition, he offers probably the only long-term solution to dietary control. Peter continues to practice in the UK.